Adrenal Reset Diet

The Ultimate Beginner's Guide To Adrenal Fatigue Reset Diet - Naturally Reset Hormones, Reduce Stress & Anxiety and Boost Your Energy Levels

By *Louise Jiannes*

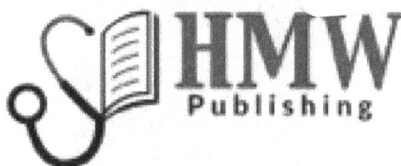

I0136184

HMW Publishing

For more great books visit:

HMWPublishing.com

Download another book for Free

I want to thank you for purchasing this book and offer you another book (just as long and valuable as this book), "Health & Fitness Mistakes You Don't Know You're Making", completely free.

Visit the link below to signup and receive it:

www.hmwpublishing.com/gift

In this book, I will break down the most common health & fitness mistakes, you are probably committing right now, and I will reveal how you can easily get in the best shape of your life!

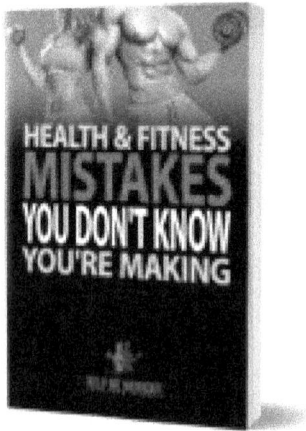

In addition to this valuable gift, you will also have an opportunity to get our new books for free, enter giveaways, and receive other valuable emails from me. Again, visit the link to sign up:

www.hmwpublishing.com/gift

TABLE OF CONTENTS

Introduction

I want to thank you and congratulate you for downloading the "*Adrenal Reset Diet*" book. This book contains proven steps and strategies on how to treat your tired adrenal glands and recover at home and includes everything else you need to know about adrenal fatigue. You will also discover what exactly causes exhausted adrenals and how your day-to-day habits and diet overwork your adrenal glands. Moreover, you will learn how getting enough sleep, avoiding stress and stressors, and being aware of the foods that you are sensitive to will help you recover and promote healthier adrenals. Likewise, this book will also explain and reveal how you can get better quality rest and sleep, the best diet for adrenal diet, and how to deal with stress to aid you in your recovery. Lastly, this book will also provide the best test options that you can choose from to find out if you really do have adrenal fatigue!

Also, before you get started, I recommend you **joining our email newsletter** to receive updates on any upcoming new book releases or promotions. You can sign-up for free, and as a bonus, you will receive a free gift. Our "*Health & Fitness Mistakes You Don't Know You're Making*" book! This book has been written to demystify, expose the top do's and don'ts and to finally equip you with the information you need to get in the best shape of your life. Due to the overwhelming amount of mis-information and lies told by magazines and self-proclaimed "gurus", it's becoming harder and harder to get reliable information to get in shape. As opposed to having to go through dozens of biased, unreliable and un-trustworthy sources to get your health & fitness information. Everything you need to help you has been broken down in this book for you to easily follow and to immediately get results to achieve your desired fitness goals in the shortest amount of time.

Once again, to join our free email newsletter and to receive a free copy of this valuable book, please visit the link and signup now: www.hmwpublishing.com/gift

CHAPTER 1: WHAT IS ADRENAL FATIGUE?

If you are like me, then the discovery of adrenal fatigue will be quite a surprise to you, and the importance of the adrenal glands is unknown. However, the fact that you are reading this book is the first step to start improving your overall health.

What are the adrenal glands?

Their names are directly related to their location, "ad" – meaning at or near and "renes" meaning kidney, which, in combination, means near the kidney. The adrenal glands are two small structures on top of each kidney. These are triangular-shaped and each measure about 3 inches long and 1 1/2 inches high. They may be small, but they play a huge and essential part in the overall health of the body. They release chemicals called hormones into the bloodstream, which affects many parts of the body, especially during the times of stress.

The adrenal glands are made up of two distinct parts that produce hormones the body needs

The Adrenal Cortex

This is the outer part of the gland, and it produces hormones that are vital to life, such as:

Cortisol

- Helps your body respond to stress and regulate metabolism,

- Stimulate the production of glucose by mobilizing free fatty acids and amino acids, and

- Have significant anti-inflammatory effects

Aldosterone

- Helps control blood pressure by maintaining the body's water and salt levels. Without the aldosterone, your kidney will lose excessive amounts of sodium (salt), consequently, water, which will lead to severe dehydration.

Testosterone and dehydroepiandrosterone (DHEA)

- These are male sex hormones, and they are involved in creating and then maintaining the differences between men and women. They have weak effects in the body, but they play a vital role in the development of male sex organs in childhood and also I women during puberty.

The Adrenal Medulla

This is the inner part of the gland, and it produces the nonessential hormones or hormones that you do not need to live, such as the **adrenaline,** small amounts of **dopamine,** and **noradrenaline**, which also helps the body react to emotional or physical stress. This may be the first thing that will come to your mind when the adrenal gland is mentioned. In your science class, you may remember your teacher or professor talking about the fight or flight response, wherein the body prepared itself to spring into action during a stressful situation. That feeling you get during exciting situations is the work of your adrenal glands, like when a person being able to carry a heavy object during a fire. The hormones secreted optimize your survival capabilities, allowing your body to respond more efficiently and effectively.

You may know adrenaline by its other name, epinephrine, which increases the rush of blood to your brain and muscles and your heart rate. It also increases the level of sugar in your body, helping the liver convert glycogen into glucose. On the other hand, noradrenaline or norepinephrine can cause vasoconstriction or narrowing of blood vessels, which leads to high blood pressure.

At the same time, **when your body is not under extreme stress, the adrenal glands are silently working to maintain your body's health**.

What Causes Adrenal Fatigue Syndrome?

As its name implies, adrenal fatigue occurs when your adrenal glands are tired –they are unable to keep up with daily needs demand your body requires of them. When the

adrenal glands are exhausted, your body will feel its effect –
you will most likely feel tired, too.

As mentioned, they produce various hormones that the body
needs and influences how your body metabolize fat, deal
with physical and emotional stress, and regulate blood sugar.

However, when your body's demand is higher than what
your adrenal system can produce and if you do not take care
of your adrenal glands as they deserve, that is when your
body's health starts declining – your body will accurately
reflect the condition of your adrenal glands.

The Fight of Fight Response

The adrenal glands are continually responding to physical
and emotional stimuli to deliver a suitable response to the
situations you are experiencing. The adrenal glands
continuously regulate the production of necessary hormones
during every condition.

If you haven't eaten all day, the cortisol regulators will tell
your body to hang on to fat because your body is not getting
enough food or fuel and maybe you will need to conserve fat

to live on. When you eat sugary food, the cortisol will surge the insulin production of your body to deal with what you just ate.

Everything you experience and do affects your adrenal glands. **If your body is continually dealing with extremes, then your adrenal glands will become exhausted and stressed, thus, leading to an adrenal fatigue syndrome**.

Is Adrenal Fatigue Syndrome the same as Chronic Fatigue Syndrome?

Adrenal fatigue syndrome is also sometimes referred to as chronic adrenal fatigue, which can lead to some confusion. Chronic fatigue syndrome and adrenal fatigue syndrome do have similar symptoms, but they have different causes. However, there is indeed a relationship between adrenal fatigue and chronic fatigue - adrenal fatigue syndrome is often present in cases of chronic fatigue syndrome. Hence, employing changes that will recharge and support your adrenal glands should be a part of the plan when managing chronic fatigue syndrome.

Do I Have Adrenal Fatigue Syndrome?

If you've experienced a nervous breakdown in the past or heard the of the term used to describe what someone is suffering, then you will have an idea of the symptoms of adrenal fatigue syndrome. Both have similar symptoms. In fact, a person's inability to cope with stress is not caused by the breakdown of nerves. It is caused by tired adrenal glands, which burn out after long periods of extreme stress and situations.

Symptoms of Adrenal Fatigue Syndrome

If you are experiencing any of the following symptoms below, it may be high time to give your adrenal glands the recharging they need.

- **Easily startled**

  If something as the ringing of a phone causes your heart to pound wildly in your chest?

- **Always feeling tired**

  Do you wake up feeling tired even after a good night's sleep? Do you take a nap during the day, but you feel like you haven't rested at all?

- **Allergies**

  Have you recently developed new allergies? Have you experienced an increase in the severity of the allergic reaction, even including anaphylaxis?

- **Increase in panic attacks or anxiety/ Diminished ability to cope with stress**

  Do you feel yourself unraveling? Do you feel unable to deal with things? Are you easily irritated? Do you feel anxious and overwhelmed?

- **Postural Hypotension**

  Do you feel dizzy after rising, especially after getting up from lying down?

- **Lethargy**

  Do you feel helplessly weak, mainly because you are not eating regularly?

- **Hypoglycemia**

  Is your blood sugar level low?

- **Hypotension**

  Is your blood pressure low?

- **Hypothyroid**

  Are you experiencing low thyroid? This usually accompanies reduced adrenal gland function.

- **Caffeine dependent**

  Do you need caffeinated drinks to start and keep going during the day?

- **Weight gain**

  Is there an increase in your weight? Do you notice that you are not losing any weight no matter what you try? Is there an increase in the amount of fat in your belly area?

- **Sensitivity to bright light**

  Are you having a hard time driving, especially during at night?

- **Disruption in sleep pattern**

  Do you feel the need to sleep in? Do you get your best sleep between 7 to 9 am? Does your body need time to get going and then become energetic all of the sudden? Does your productivity decrease during the late afternoon and you feel the need to take a nap? Are you tired during the early hours of the evening, but not able to sleep early? Do you feel energized after 11 pm and can get going until early in the morning? This unhealthy sleeping pattern will usually make you feel tired the next day.

* **Unable to recuperate or fight off illness**
Do you often feel sick all the time?

* **Does exercise make you feel worse, not better?**

* **Low libido**
Do you have little to no interest or energy for sex? Do you experience a weird, hit your funny bone, raw nerve pain feeling during orgasm? Does orgasm make you fell wipe-out or jittery, but not in a good way.

* **Food cravings**
Do you often crave for sweet, salty, and protein-rich food?

- **Multiple stress or continual stress factors**

  Did you just have a baby, got married, had surgery, got divorced, moved to another town or country, lost a loved one, have 3 kids under 5, have tweens, have teens, been a victim of a crime, lost a job, have a job, or any kind of situation that gives your stress? Stress factors do not necessarily mean adverse situations or conditions, and they do not have to be dramatic. Stress factors can be something continual – all the little stressors you experience can add up and cause adrenal fatigue.

The symptoms mentioned above are often ignored when you look at them individually. But when you see them as pieces of the same puzzle, they spell out adrenal gland fatigue syndrome, which means that you need to give your glands tender loving care.

CHAPTER 2: CAN I TEST MY ADRENAL FUNCTION AT HOME?

You may feel like you have adrenal fatigue syndrome, but you want to make sure. Then there are tests that you can do at home.

Postural Hypotension

This test is also known as orthostatic hypotension. It's a drop in blood pressure that happens when a person rises from lying down. If you ever experience what people often refer to us head rush, lightheadedness, feeling of dizziness, or standing up too fast, then you would be familiar with this.

For this test, you will need a blood pressure cuff. Lie down and rest for about 5 minutes. Measure your blood pressure while you are lying down, and then stand up and measure your blood pressure again.

Typically, blood pressure should rise about 10-20 points. If your blood pressure drops by 10 points or more, it indicates hypoadrenia. The more significant the drop in blood pressure, the greater the adrenal insufficiency.

It is also important to mention that in general, a low blood pressure usually indicates exhausted adrenal, particularly when you have the other symptoms of adrenal gland fatigue.

Iris Contraction Test

To do this test, you will need a mirror and a weak penlight or flashlight. Go into a dark closet or bathroom and wait for a couple of minutes to let your eyes to adjust to the darkness – this will allow the pupils of your eyes to dilate or fully open. Then shine the penlight or flashlight into your eyes, and through the mirror, watch the reaction of your pupils for at least 30 minutes.

The light should cause the iris of your eyes to contract, making your pupils or the darker spot in the center of your eyes to become smaller. Usually, the pupils should stay small. If you have adrenal gland fatigue, the pupils will be weak, and they will not hold the contraction, and they will waver between relaxed and contracted, or, it will initially contract, but then expand after 10 to 30 seconds.

The weaker the ability of the pupils to contract indicates the weakness of your adrenal glands.

Sergent's Adrenal White Line

Using the dull end of a spoon or your fingernail, draw a line across your belly. When you have a moderate to severe case of adrenal fatigue, the line will stay white and, in some cases, become wider over time. Usually, the line would almost immediately turn red.

Historically, this test has been used to indicate severe adrenal fatigue and Addison's disease. If you have a milder case of adrenal fatigue, the test may not show any sign.

24-Hour Adrenal Hormone Saliva Test

An Adrenal Function Test (Full Day Cortisol + DHEA) test is the best way to find out the state or condition of the adrenal function.

Adrenal Function Test (Full Day Cortisol + DHEA)

To do this test, you can directly order a test kit from the laboratory, or you can ask your doctor to provide you with a kit that you can take home and complete. For this test, you will have to collect a small sample of your saliva in a small vial 4 times a day during specific hours – around 7 am, 11 am, 4 pm, and finally 11 pm. After you collect the 4 samples, you will need to mail the kit for analysis in a laboratory. The test will cost about 175 dollars, including the cost of the kit and the analysis. The results of the analysis will typically come out after 5 to 7 days and will usually be e-mailed to you. For an additional fee, you can also schedule a consultation with the lab's staff physician to review the results with you.

Saliva Test versus Blood Tests

Although cortisol hormone levels can be measured using blood tests, results from saliva tests are far more superior. Blood tests often measure both the active and inactive forms of the hormone. Usually, the result will look as if your body is making enough hormones when in reality there is not enough. For testing for adrenal fatigue, you will need to focus on the level of active adrenal hormones.

The level of cortisol in the body fluctuates in a particular pattern during the day. Taking 4 samples will help your doctor see if the level is dropping and spiking at the correct hours. Some tests will include measuring the levels of dehydroepiandrosterone sulfate or DHEA-S, the male hormone, androgen created in the adrenal glands, and graph the relationship between cortisol and DHEA.

If you think that you have adrenal fatigue, then the most efficient and helpful way is to have the test results with you when you first visit your doctor for a consultation. This way, your doctor will have as much information to start with. Otherwise, you will leave the doctor's office will most likely an instruction to run some tests to find out what you are dealing with.

How Do I Interpret Home Hormone Test Kit Results?

Most companies will offer some summary of the cortisol level test results when you order a test kit, noting the normal range. Here are some of the things you need to keep in mind when you are interpreting the results of your test.

- The cortisol cycle follows the circadian rhythm of your body.

- The level of cortisol is highest in the morning to help you wake up and get ready for the day.

- It lowers during the day and then rises again after you have eaten – this is why it's vital to eat frequently because it helps keeps blood sugar more stable, thus, making your cortisol level more stable.

- The cortisol levels in your body should be at their lowest at night, allowing you to sleep.

- If you force your body to stay awake, particularly later in the evening, it will lead to the release of cortisol, which will keep you from falling asleep, requiring your adrenal glands to produce more cortisol as it responds to stress. This will be especially hard on your adrenals because they need to rest overnight to recharge and ready for the next day.

- Work shifts are particularly hard on your adrenal glands because it continually demands them to change their natural pattern of cortisol production. Moreover, our body will never entirely get accustomed to because it goes against the flow, particularly if you are keeping a daytime schedule on the weekends or you have frequently worked in alternate shifts.

- When your adrenal glands weaken, they lose their ability to regulate themselves and will overproduce in the early stages of adrenal fatigue. Imagine a wagon going downhill. It will seem that the adrenal glands are working too well, but in fact, this is the adrenal gland finally burning out and can no longer produce sufficient cortisol –they are actually exhausted to regulate themselves.

What are the "Normal Ranges" of Cortisol Level Test Results?

Adrenal fatigue and low thyroid, its common companion, are conditions that are often hard to quantify by tests alone. The best way to diagnose is treating the presence of classic symptoms until the symptoms abate. Why? Because the normal range of the test results is extensive – your result can show half of someone else's and still be considered normal. If your results are on the low end of normal, then there is still a lot of room for improvement. Moreover, if you do not have a test result during a time when you felt better, then your first test result may not be even "normal" for you. What if you used to be at the high end of normal when you felt better? If your level dropped by 25, 30, or 50 percent, it wouldn't matter if it falls into the official "normal range, it is still not normal for you.

For example, the 8 am "normal" range 3.5 to 6.3 means that you could have nearly HALF as much or conversely TWICE as much and you will still be within the normal range. Likewise, the test results can be dramatically different during different days, so your results during a stressful day can be very different.

The interesting fact about the adrenal glands is that they can recharge and repair themselves when you are lying down, and their prime healing is between 7-9 am. So if you feel like sleeping in late, then do so – it's a very part of your adrenal glands recovery process.

Sometimes, letting yourself do the things your body is asking to could be the hardest part. However, acknowledging that you have a problem is the first step to recovery. This is no different when you have adrenal fatigue syndrome. If you continue to push through with the fatigue, it will only make the condition worse. So rest and sleep when you need to, don't skimp on it.

Do I Really Need a Saliva Cortisol Test?

This is a debated topic. Some people who are familiar with adrenal fatigue don't always see taking a saliva test necessary to diagnose and treat adrenal fatigue cases, particularly those of mild to moderate.

On the other hand, the results of the test could reveal useful information and provide evidence that will support a diagnosis for cases when symptoms alone do not give a clear picture. Moreover, it can help determine if your symptoms are from adrenal fatigue, where the glands produce too much cortisol or if your condition has progressed to the point where the body is not creating sufficient cortisol or a more advanced form of adrenal fatigue.

Additionally, a test will reveal the pattern of your cortisol levels throughout the day – if it differs or follow the optimal pattern and it relates to your symptoms throughout the day.

Of course, this is only a snapshot of one day. Depending on your stress levels, how well you slept, etc., the results can vary from day to day. By its own, the test alone won't be able to tell you if you have adrenal fatigue. But it does provide evidence to be considered, together with your symptoms, and possibly, along with other tests to assess the function of your thyroid as well the other hormones – testosterone, progesterone, and estrogen.

Do I Need a Doctor to Order my Saliva Cortisol Test?

Many people with adrenal fatigue syndrome do not have doctors who are familiar with the condition, so most of them take matters into their own hands. Hence, they are most likely to order a cortisol test themselves.

Every case is different. You may have a different level of knowledge and comfort as far as taking charge of your health and understanding of your condition. Most of the time, taking the test is just one way to confirm what you know all along – that there is indeed something causing your problems. You may need it for peace of mind.

You can always opt to see a doctor first before taking the test – it may be covered by insurance if ordered through their lab or office. However, in most cases, adrenal fatigue is not recognized as a valid diagnosis and will refuse to pay for the test. Every situation is different and it really up to you and your diligence to decide on what is the best course of action.

Whichever the case is for you, the collection of the sample saliva will still be done by you at home and the samples mailed to the lab. However, you will want to take advantage of the turnaround of the results. If you order the test online, you can get the results within two weeks, compared to the 2 months or more by getting a doctor's appointment, for the test, taking the test, and then another appointment to go over the results. As mentioned earlier, it can be advantageous to have test results the first time you visit the doctor – it can be more productive.

In short, there are available tests that you can order online, but it is up to you to decide which course of action to take.

Remember, you can begin making changes even before you decide to take the test. Learning more about adrenal fatigue syndrome and making changes in your lifestyle to support your adrenal glands and reducing stress is the key to feeling better. Even if adrenal fatigue is not your primary diagnosis, your adrenal glands play an important role in your health. Making changes to help their recovery will significantly benefit you.

CHAPTER 3: STRESS AND LACK OF SLEEP AFFECTS YOUR ADRENAL GLANDS

You know by now the adrenal fatigue is a stress-related and sleep-related condition. In this chapter, let's take a close look at the kinds of stress and how sleep affects our adrenal glands.

What Is "Stress"?

Since our adrenal glands are in charge of how our bodies respond to stress, they affect the function of our adrenal, one way or another. In this manner, let's take a look at the many types of stress that can affect our lives and our adrenal glands.

Usually, when we talk about stress, we often refer to emotional or mental stress – the things we recognize, and we know as needing an immediate reaction, finances, children, workplace issues, etc. However, there are other types of stress, environmental and physical factors, what we do not realize that are stressing the adrenal system.

The combination of environmental and physical stressors is usually what affects the production of hormones in our adrenal glands, which lead to adrenal fatigue. Sleep, for instance, is caused by both physical and environmental factors.

Nevertheless, it is important to keep in mind that not all stress is negative. Even happy occasions can be stressful to your adrenals. Planning a wedding, getting married, pregnancy, having children, and landing a job, etc. can also cause stress, despite the fact that these events are exciting and you will even look forward to them.

Below are some of the physical and chemical stressors that can affect the adrenal glands.

Physical stress
- Alcohol and caffeine consumption

- Chronic pain

- Illness

- Inadequate sleep

- Mineral and vitamin deficiencies

- Noise

- Obesity

- Poor diet

- Pregnancy

- Smoking

- Surgery

- Systemic yeast infections

Chemical stress

- Bug sprays

- Fluorescent lighting

- Fluoridated/chlorinated water

- Household cleaning chemicals

- Medications/drugs, especially corticosteroids

- New carpet

- Plastics

- Workplace or home air pollution

- Yard chemicals

How Does Stress Affect Health?

As stress remains continuously high or increases, the adrenal glands work overtime to deal with the situation or condition. During these times, you may find yourself craving for caffeine and sugar to help maintain alertness. You are doing precisely the wrong thing – you create an even greater demand on your adrenals. This short-term relief will eventually do your body more harm than good.

At the same time, contact to hidden adrenal stressors, such as exposure to chemicals, weakens your adrenals. Hence, your glands are not able to respond optimally – you are losing the battlefront on this one.

When the many and dramatic physical stressors continue for a long time, the high levels of cortisol circulating in your body can change the standard processes of your metabolic system. It hastens cell aging and causes the development of resistance to insulin and ultimately diabetes, as well as, inhibiting sleep, weight loss, and immune function. This, in turn, will cause additional stress to your adrenal glands because they will have to respond to the stress caused by lack of sleep, excess weight, and illness.

How Am I Supposed to Avoid Things that are Stressful?

Realistically, you will not be able to eliminate everything that causes stress in your life. It's not even advisable – some stress is actually beneficial!

The key is to be aware of your stress, good and bad, and to learn which stressors to avoid and eliminate and which ones you need to learn to manage better. Creating a healthy lifestyle will help reduce the on your adrenals.

Sufficient Sleep and Stress Relief Helps the Adrenal Gland Recover

One of the most important and the very first thing that you need to start recharging your adrenal is sleep. Most of the time, you will find it hard to sleep or sleep at the right times when you have adrenal fatigue.

How Can I Get Enough Sleep?

What do you do when you feel sleepy in the afternoon? Do you push yourself through the need to sleep and often pump it up with coffee or tea? This habit always triggers a response to stress from your adrenal glands.

Allow yourself to sleep as much as you can, even if it's in the middle of the day. When you feel groggy, it's your adrenals telling you that they need a break. So lay down on a sofa and put your feet up for a couple of minutes. Lying horizontally, even it is only for 15 minutes, will do your adrenals some good.

If you can, sleep in in the mornings, especially when you are feeling particularly tired. If you have to drop your kids off to school, then go back to bed as soon as you can. Some of the vital rechargings of your adrenals happen between 7 to 9 in the morning.

The more you let your body to see when it wants to, the faster your body will be able to recover, up to a point where you will not need to sleep at inconvenient times.

Stick to a sleep schedule. Plan to be in bed no later than between 9 to 9:45 in the evening. Sleep is crucial to adrenal gland repair. You need to sleep as regularly as you can, especially when you are in the intensive rebuilding phase.

Cortisol and Sleep

Earlier, we've tackled about cortisol as one of the stress-response hormones that the adrenal glands produce. Lack of good-quality sleep or lack of sleep affects the cortisol levels in your system, but not in the manner that you probably think. You would think that when you are tired, the levels of cortisol will drop, right? However, when you don't get sufficient sleep, your body actually releases more cortisol for extended periods of time.

Usually, cortisol levels are at their highest in the mornings and decreases by nighttime. During the day, your body will release extra cortisol throughout the day to respond to any physical or emotional stress.

When your body has too much cortisol at night, it will keep you from sleeping deeply, you will wake up frequently during the night, and you will wake up feeling unrested.

This leads to a vicious cycle – the lack of restful and deep sleep itself is a stressor, causing your adrenals to release more cortisol, which in turn, will prevent you from getting the rest and sleep you need to stop the cycle.

Why Am I So Tired All the Time?

Stressor number one - you force yourself to wake up and start the day earlier than your body wants to. You are starting on the wrong foot. When you have adrenal fatigue syndrome, your body's most restful and deep sleep comes between 6:00-9:00 am – right around the time most of us would usually be waking up and getting ready for the day. So even if you feel tired and unrested, you force yourself to wake up, get up, and get going. When you are doing this, you are stressing your adrenal glands, which the first stress-induced cortisol release of the day.

Stressor number two – to wake yourself up, you drink a cup of coffee. If you are like many people, then your day officially starts after a sip of morning Joe. Otherwise, you are cranky and unsociable. Most of us also start the day with pancakes, a muffin, toast, cereal, etc. for breakfast. These are all foods that are packed with simple carbohydrates that quickly turn to sugar, which triggers the cortisol to release its second stress-induced release for the day to help balance the levels of insulin and blood sugar in your body.

Stressor number three – the struggle of your daily morning routine. It's particularly stressful when you have young children. You have to help them wake up and get up, bath them, dress them, fed them, search for lost socks, find lost homework – they need to be ready before the bus arrives or you have to get things going before you need to go to work.

Stressor number four, five, six... - if you are working parent, a challenging day at work only adds to your stress. By the time you get to the office, your heart is pumping, and the adrenaline rush has completely worked you up and got you going. By 10 in the morning, your body experiences a blood sugar crash, which you set up eating a meal packed with simple carbs, so you will take another cup of coffee to get your body going until lunchtime. More blood sugar and caffeine roller-coaster stressors.

After lunchtime, you will feel the need to take a nap, but what will other people say? Sleeping at work, or even at home, in the middle of the day seems like something only a lazy person will do. So you push through, probably with another cup of coffee, which leads to yet another stress-hormone release. You force yourself to work even though your brain isn't functioning well anymore and it no longer thinks clearly – things will probably be hazy.

By the time that all of the day's work is done, you are feeling so tired, and you no longer have energy, so you probably decide to get dinner from the drive-through on the way home or just make something easy to eat when you get back home. You probably can't wait for bedtime by this hour.

Finally, by the time your kids are in bed, around 9:00 pm, you lay in bed looking forward to rest, but you can't relax. Your heart and mind are still racing, but you can't relax and fall asleep even though you feel so tired. You have been dragging all afternoon, but you can't sleep. You lay in bed, tossing and turning for 2-3 hours because the levels of cortisol in your body are still high. You start feeling anxious because it's already 1:00 am, and you are not asleep yet, and you will have to get up again soon – you need to sleep, but you are missing it.

And those are just your typical, everyday routine stressors. You may have to top those stressors with a new boss, a new job, a new baby, a wedding, a death of a loved one, a fender-bender, volunteer or employment obligations, interpersonal conflict, etc.

What Do I Need to Do to Solve my Problem?

The very first thing that you need to do is **to start listening to the signals your body is giving you – when you need to sleep, stop ignoring it**. Sleep in. Take a nap. Stop feeling guilty. It's not being lazy. Resist the urge to stay up late because you have a good second wind – that energetic feeling at night is actually a reversed cortisol cycle, the levels peaking at night instead of in the morning.

To help stop the vicious cycle, listen to your body. Nap or sleep whenever your body is asking to. Resting and sleeping whenever your body will help you get deeper sleep cycles, restore your adrenal glands, and reduce the cortisol released by stress caused by sleep deprivation. In turn, this will help reduce the overall levels of cortisol in your body during bedtime, making it easier for you to sleep at night.

Listen to your body. Do not worry about developing a bad sleeping schedule. Your health is compromised, and you need rest and sleep for your adrenal treatment and recovery. Taking 500 grams of magnesium at bedtime will help your body physically relax, and Gamma-Amino Butyric acid (GABA), an amino acid that inhibits nerve transmission in the brain will help you mentally relax.

CHAPTER 4: IS THERE A CURE FOR ADRENAL FATIGUE?

That is the question. Often, when people ask it, what they usually mean is, "What can I take to make me feel better by next week? However, curing adrenal fatigue syndrome is not as simple as popping pills.

Adrenal fatigue is a condition caused by lifestyle and merely taking medication isn't going to cure the underlying problems behind it. Everyone's adrenal exhaustion is slightly different from one to the other, so no single answer will cure it. To address your adrenal fatigue adequately, you will need to identify your stressors and decide on how to modify or eliminate those stressors. The key to your recovery is to find solutions that fit your unique adrenal fatigue problem.

If your adrenal fatigue is caused predominantly by sensitivity to food, then it will be helpful to take an adrenal glandular. However, it will never truly be resolved until the food that causes your fatigue are identified and removed from your diet.

If your job is the source of your stress, then practicing relaxation breathing techniques only acts as a bandage to a large wound. You may need to think and consider getting a different job. You may want to try working at home or search for a low-stress job.

If your adrenal glands are tired because of constant stressors, such as caring for a terminally ill or elderly family member, then it's likely that you have pushed aside caring for yourself. If this is your case, then the plan for your treatment will need to include getting better sleep, eating better, and having someone to talk to about your feeling, aside from taking adrenal supplements for your recovery.

The adrenal fatigue treatment for you will be different from the treatment of your friend. To unlock your personalized treatment plan, then you need to identify the causes of your adrenal fatigue. While a doctor can help you with diagnosis and developing a plan for your treatment, you are your own best healthcare provider. It is up to you to understand your condition, address the causes, and make changes in your life that will help restore your health.

REDUCE and REBUILD: How to Treat Adrenal Exhaustion

There are two approaches to successfully recover and treat from adrenal exhaustion:

1. **Reducing the stressors that are exhausting your adrenal glands**, and;

2. **Rebuilding your adrenal glands**

To do that, you need to address and change three (3) separate changes in your lifestyle for healthy living.

- Nutrition and Diet,

- Sleep, and,

- Stress Reduction

Each of those areas has some specific and essential DONT's and DO's to treat adrenal fatigue.

Reduce the Stressors that Cause Adrenal Exhaustion

Nutrition/Diet

With the goal of completely removing food that raises blood sugar and stimulates over-production of cortisol, such as artificial sweeteners, sugar, allergens, and caffeine, you will need to start reducing the amount your consumption of the foods mentioned above.

Quitting substances like caffeine can be as stressful on your adrenal glands as drinking them. So don't go cold turkey right away. Begin by reducing your everyday consumption by half.

Sleep

Waking up early, ignoring the urge to rest and nap, and staying up late at night stresses your adrenals, which need to repair themselves at night when you sleep. So sleep as much as your body needs. It's not selfish. It's not being lazy, and it's not optional. In fact, getting the sleep your body needs is very important for your treatment and recovery. It will influence the length of your recovery time. If you don't get as much sleep as your body needs, it will shorten your treatment time.

Get out of the vicious cycle. Stop drinking caffeinated drinks to stay awake and stop taking pills to help you sleep. There artificial "downers" and "uppers" negatively influence your adrenal signals, cortisol cycle, and circadian rhythm and harm your body.

The best way to have enough energy to start the day is to get enough deep and restful sleep, not coffee. You can take an adrenal glandular supplement to help raise the levels of your cortisol in the morning where you really need them and taking a magnesium supplement before sleep will help you relax and sleep, and help support the recovery of your adrenal function.

Stress Reduction

To reduce your stressors, you will first need to **identify the relationships or situations that high levels of stress**. Make a list of the things in your life that makes it very stressful. This will include not only the big things. It should also include the little things such as the constant dripping of a kitchen faucet that needs fixing could that gets on your nerves. The small stuff may not be the leading cause of your adrenal exhaustion, but the little things that irritate and cause you to worry can add up and keep you from getting downtime to relax.

Second, eliminate the environmental toxins, such as plastics, fluoride, chlorine, and other endocrine disruptors. Watch out for common household cleaners that you are exposed to and often use. Most of these chemicals are highly toxic and dangerous and should be eliminated from your home. They contribute to your adrenal exhaustion.

Finally, moderate your physical activity. While exercise is good for the health, excessive physical exertion drains your adrenal glands. Choose a light exercise, yoga, walking, etc. over fast-paced aerobic workout.

Rebuild your Adrenal Glands

Nutrition/Diet

Follow the **Adrenal Fatigue Diet and Guidelines** tackled in the next chapter about the right way of eating: high protein, three (3) meals, and three (3) snacks.

Taking supplements is also a vital part when you are treating and recovering from adrenal exhaustion. You can consider taking care vitamin B-complex, vitamin C, high-quality multivitamin, GABA, magnesium, and adrenal glandular.

Sleep

You have learned the connection between lack of restful, deep sleep and stress relief in the earlier chapters. As mentioned, do not sleep later than 9:00-10:00 pm and stick to it. Stay in bed as late as you can, as often as you can. Your adrenal glands repair themselves best between 7:00-9:00 am. When you need to do something in the morning, go back to sleep as soon as you can.

Take a rest and nap when your body tells you. When you fight to stay awake when you are sleepy, you are putting a demand on your adrenal glands to function beyond their capacity. Plan a nap between your daily activities.

Stress Reduction

Create a plan to deal, reduce, and eliminate with stressful relationships and situations. Take the time to examine the source of your stresses and brainstorm a plan to deal with each one.

Is there a way that you can remove or solve the source of this stress? If not, how can you reduce it? You can probably check off a couple of little stressors from the list quickly. Other stressors will not be resolved promptly. Taking time to identify these stressors and considering solutions is in itself therapeutic. You might even actually come up with a workable solution.

You can also learn some relaxation breathing exercises ad practices. You can use them to relax whenever you feel anxious. It's a great way to re-train your body's stress response.

Several herbs that can help reduce stress. Aromatherapy, such as lavender, herbal tea, such as chamomile, and nutritional supplement, such as Valerian, can help relieve stress.

The cause of adrenal fatigue is different for everyone, so your approach to treating and recovering from adrenal exhaustion must be personal and fit your situation. Identify your weak spots, make a plan to reduce or eliminate stressors, and make the needed changes in your lifestyle for treatment and recovery.

CHAPTER 5: THE ADRENAL FATIGUE DIET AND GUIDELINES FOR TREATMENT AND RECOVERY

What foods should I be eating when I have adrenal fatigue? What foods bring me more harm than good? For adrenal exhaustion treatment and recovery, here are the DON'T's and DO's that you need to follow.

The essential diet for a person with adrenal fatigue is similar to any healthy lifestyle diet. Your meals should consist of nutritious, high-quality food that will help keep the levels of blood sugar in your body stable to maintain healthy adrenal function.

You probably have been eating meals that directly affect the function of your adrenal glands, or worse, skipping meals, which is also hard on them. Coffee and other caffeinated drinks, food packed with artificial sweeteners, unhealthy meals, and unhealthy eating patterns hinder the recovery of your adrenal glands.

Eat frequent, high-protein 3 meals and 3 snacks every day.

Eat your breakfast 30 minutes after you wake up and plan to eat high protein recipes every 2 to 3 hours to help keep the levels of your blood sugar stable.

Eat "REAL" food.

When shopping food for your meals, avoid pre-packaged mixes and any imitation pasteurized processed cheese. Avoid canned and instant food. Avoid anything that you won't have to cook yourself. These foods are packed with preservatives and other additives that can hinder the function of your adrenal glands. Always choose fresh or frozen produce, vegetables, fruits, meat, etc.

Forget you know about "breakfast foods."

The worst things you can eat for breakfast are sugar-rich food, such as cereals and fruits. These foods quickly turn to sugar and spike the level of your blood sugar, which, in turn, will make your adrenals work harder to catch up when you crash later in the morning.

Think of protein-rich food instead.

Meat and eggs are the best foods to start your day. If you choose to eat fruit, then decide to eat whole fruits, which are high in fiber, which helps absorb sugar. Avoid drinking fruit juices in the morning, which just gives your body a sugar jolt. If you do choose fruit, then follow it up 30 minutes later with something more substantial.

If you must eat grain products, avoid white flour and white sugar. Choose whole-grain options, such as pumpernickel toast and oatmeal, which are complex carbohydrates that take longer to metabolize. And, of course, include some protein. An easy and quick breakfast option is a delicious, protein meal shake.

Limit sugary and starchy fruits and vegetables.

Bananas, in particular, are high in potassium, which causes adrenal fatigue. As often as possible, choose non-starchy vegetables. Lightly cooked or raw are the best preparation options. However, if you are using crucifers, such as cauliflower, cabbage, and broccoli, make sure to cook them always - this neutralizes goitrogenic compounds, which are thyroid suppressors.

Eliminate white flours and white sugar.

Simple carbohydrates require greater amounts of insulin. It makes it harder for your adrenal glands to stabilize the levels of sugar in your body, hence, stressing them.

Always choose whole-grain options. Complex carbohydrates make you feel fuller faster, slower to digest, provide fiber, and takes longer to process, thus, moderating the levels of blood sugar in your body.

If you want to sweeten your food, use raw honey, palm sugar, or Xylitol.

Avoid "diet" food.

The word diet in food products does not mean that they are healthy for you. Diet sodas, for example, are packed with artificial sweeteners. Non-fat food products that should actually have some fat in them will wreak havoc not just on people with adrenaline fatigue, but also to everyone in general. Artificial fats and artificial sweeteners should not be considered a part of a healthy diet. In fact, these foods can actually cause weight gain.

Completely eliminate caffeine.

This is easier said and done. If you are used to pumping your body with coffee or with caffeinated drinks to keep you going throughout the day, then it will take getting used to. Quitting and drinking coffee is both hard on your adrenal glands. As mentioned earlier, if you are a coffee addict, gradually wean yourself. Cut your daily consumption in half, and then again, in half.

Completely eliminate alcohol.

Like caffeine, alcohol is a tricky substance to eliminate, and you can't just go cold turkey. Slowly reduce your consumption until you have successfully removed it from your diet. If you have adrenal fatigue and you are having a hard time stabilizing blood sugar, the book Potatoes Not Prozac: Solutions for Sugar Sensitivity discusses the connection between sugar sensitivity and alcohol cravings, along with a 7-step plan to control sugar cravings.

Do NOT limit your salt intake.

When you have adrenal fatigue, you will be craving for something salty. Sodium is important for adrenal gland function. When your adrenals are exhausted, they are usually low in sodium. However, not all salts are created equal. Celtic Sea Salt is an abundant source of trace minerals, aside from sodium, which makes it a healthier salt. Another good choice is Himalayan pink salt, which is excellent in a shaker. Sea salt and Himalayan salt have different salt mineral contents so one may make you feel better than the other. You can keep both on hand – use sea salt for recipes and use Himalayan salt as a shaker on the table. Variety is indeed the spice of life.

Do NOT restrict fats in your diet.

We are not talking about just any fats here. I am referring to the right kind of fats. Your body uses cholesterol and fats to make hormones. If you are not getting enough of them, then your body will not be able to produce the hormones it needs.

This is contrary to the diet trends. However, a low-fat diet actually contributes to adrenal fatigue, especially if you deprive yourself even of the healthy fats. Include good fats in your diet, such as coconut oil and grapeseed oil, both of which you can use for high heat cooking, like frying, real organic butter, and olive oil.

Identify and eliminate foods that you are sensitive and allergic to.

Food sensitivities and delayed food allergies more common than you think and the most common suspects are in the foods that you eat every day, such as corn, soy, eggs, wheat, milk, and others.

Food sensitivities and delayed food allergies may not cause dramatic reactions, such as anaphylaxis or hives, but they add to the general feeling of sickness, as well as severely stressing your adrenal glands.

Adrenal Fatigue Sample Recipes

If you are just beginning to change your diet to treat and recover from adrenal fatigue, then here are some recipes to get you started.

Adrenal Fatigue Soup a.k.a. "Taz"

This famous recipe for adrenal fatigue is high in minerals, alkalizes the system, and calming.

Ingredients:

- 1 zucchini, medium-sized, sliced

- 1 teaspoon paprika

- 1 onion, medium-sized, chopped

- 1 cup tomato juice

- 1 cup filtered water

- 1 cup chicken broth

- 1 cup celery, chopped

- 1 can (16 ounces) green beans

- 2 tablespoons raw honey

Directions:

1. Combine all of the ingredients in a stock pot and simmer for about 1 hour or until the veggies are tender.

The following 2 recipes are also great for adrenal support. The first recipe, Morning Sole, is a salt suspension that you drink in the morning. It will provide your body trace minerals that it needs for optimum cellular function.

The second recipe is a honey and salt combination you take at night. It is reported that this drink helps keep the levels of blood sugar overnight, increase the production of melatonin, and hopefully, help you sleep better.

Morning Sole

Ingredients:

- Celtic Sea Salt or Pink Himalayan Crystal Salt, enough to fill a jar 1/4 full, plus more as needed

- Water, enough to fill a jar

Equipment:

Glass jar with plastic or glass lid – do not use a metal lid.

Directions:

1. Fill the jar 1/4 full with the salt of your choice. Pour in enough water to fill the jar.

2. Let the salt dissolve overnight. If the salt is dissolved in the morning, add more salt until you reach a saturation point where no more salt is dissolved – it is okay to leave the undissolved salt in the jar. You can just add more water later when the jar gets emptier.

3. To use, scoop 1 teaspoon sole using a plastic measuring teaspoon and mix into a glass of water.

Drink this first thing in the morning before you drink or eat anything else.

Notes: Do not let any metal come in contact with the sole water.

Evening Honey and Sea Salt

Ingredients:

- 1 teaspoon raw honey

- Celtic gray sea salt or Pink Himalayan

Directions:

1. There are several versions of this recipe. Measure 1 teaspoon honey and sprinkle sea salt on top of the honey.

2. Take the mix before going to sleep.

3. Many people take a spoonful sprinkled with salt. If you have adrenal fatigue, the salt will help your adrenal glands. The proportions are not critical. Just experiment to find out what works best for your body.

Breakfast is the hardest meal if you have adrenal exhaustion. The traditional breakfast food and meal that we usually eat in the morning are not adrenal-friendly. It's already hard to start the day until you had something good to eat.

Leftover dishes from dinner are great options because they are higher in protein. The hash recipe below will take some effort to make, but it's very satisfying.

Hash-Style Breakfast

Ingredients:

- 1-2 eggs

- 1 tablespoons coconut oil, unflavored

- 1 sweet potato, medium-sized, cubed

- 1 onion, small-sized, chopped

- 1 clove garlic, crushed and then minced

- 1 beet, cubed

- Any combination of your preferred greens: kale, chard, or spinach

- Celtic sea salt, to taste

- Cremini, shiitake, Maitake, or other mushrooms of your choice

- Manchego cheese, shredded

Directions:

1. In a large-sized skillet, put the oil and heat. Add the sweet potato, beet, onion, and garlic to the skillet, and sauté until soft.

2. Add the mushrooms and toss in the greens until wilted. Season to taste with salt.

3. Crack 1-2 egg on top and cook until the egg/s is cooked to your preference. Alternatively, you can scramble the egg/s before pouring into the skillet, cooking omelet style.

4. Top with manchego cheese. Serve.

Notes: You can use either raw beet or pickled beet. If using raw, then sauté with the sweet potato until soft. If using pickled, just cube it and add it to the skillet after adding the greens, before the egg/s.

Hold your horses. Before you start cooking, read the chapter below to find out which foods you need to avoid and eliminate in your diet.

CHAPTER 6: FOOD INTOLERANCES AND DELAYED FOOD ALLERGIES CAUSE ADRENAL FATIGUE

There are hidden stressors that cause adrenal exhaustion – food intolerances and delayed food allergies. These hidden culprits may be the ones hampering your adrenal glands' recovery or any attempt to feel better. Thus, you always feel tired and unenergetic.

Usually, when the word allergy comes to mind, we typically think that in a relatively short time, we will start to see the obvious and dramatic reaction to the substances we are allergic to, such as swelling or hives and breath shortness. However, when you have delayed food allergy to a particular substance, it is not always the case. It may take hours or even days before the symptoms appear, and the symptoms may not be reactions that we recognize.

Cortisol, hormones produced by the adrenal glands, plays a vital role in responding to allergens. When you eat foods that you are allergic to frequently, your adrenal glands will continuously work to react accordingly.

When you are allergic to something as common as wheat, your adrenal glands are always on some level of alertness, and you may not even realize that food allergy is the cause of your stress.

The Difference between Food Intolerance and Food Allergy

Most of us are not aware that there are two kinds of food allergies. You could be severely allergic to something and immediately experience serious anaphylactic reactions, both of which are commonly associated with seafood and peanut allergy. This is called "true allergy" or immunoglobulin E antibodies (IgE) and is what most of us think of when people say they are allergic to something.

However, there is a second type of food allergy that is not popularly known. This food allergy is called food sensitivity, delayed food allergy, or IgG food intolerance. This food allergy is less understood, but it is far more common.

When a person has this type of food allergy, reactions and symptoms could take place after a couple of hours, even days, after eating the offending food. There are many types of reactions to this type of allergy. You may not even be aware that something you ate causes some of the physical problems you are experiencing. Who would think that something you ate 3 days ago is the culprit. Moreover, if you do associate a physical reaction to something that you ate, you would usually think it's that something unique that you ate. However, you may be allergic to something that you eat all the time. Some of the most common culprits are cow's milk, eggs, soy, peanuts, wheat, fish, tree nuts, and shellfish. Sometimes, your symptoms can be a reaction to a specific combination of food that doesn't usually cause symptoms when eaten individually.

Leaky Gut Syndrome and Adrenal Exhaustion

When a person has sensitivities to various foods, the lining of the intestines and the stomach becomes inflamed and irritated, and if the person continually eats food that irritates the digestive system, then it will not have a chance to rest and heal. This leads to heartburn, stomach pain, gas, or other discomforts. It can even lead to "Leaky Gut Syndrome," a condition which increases the penetrability of the intestine walls that allows undigested fats and proteins to "leak" out of the intestine into the bloodstream, which, in turn, causes autoimmune reactions.

When this happens, the adrenal glands are alerted to the increased levels of histamine, which causes inflammation. This, in turn, will trigger the adrenal glands to increase the secretion of cortisol, which is an anti-inflammatory.

What Does Leaky Gut Mean for People With Adrenal Gland Fatigue?

If you have adrenal fatigue and you are frequently eating food that causes autoimmune response or inflammation, then you put a significant strain on your already exhausted adrenal glands to maintain increased levels of cortisol to suppress the inflammation.

Now imagine if you are sensitive to wheat, which you eat every meal in one form or another - as an ingredient in canned soup, as a main dish like pasta, like toasted bread in the morning, or as soy sauce that you use to marinate meat in. When you have unrecognized food sensitivity, then you are continually exposing yourself to an allergen that contributes to your adrenal exhaustion.

How Can I Recognize if I Have Food Allergies?

Aside from the gastric symptoms, food sensitivity or delayed food allergy manifest themselves in symptoms you would not usually think to connect – asthma, migraines, rheumatoid arthritis, fibromyalgia and other autoimmune syndromes, autism, attention deficit disorder (ADD), and there are many more recognized as triggered by food sensitivity. People who have identified foods they are sensitive to and have eliminated them from their diets have greatly improved their health dramatically.

Delayed food allergies or food sensitivity is unknowingly the cause of many day-to-day complaints, such as:

* Acne

* Rosy cheeks

* Dark circles under the eyes

* Weight gain,

* Plugged ears

71

- Chronic ear infections

- Chronic sinus issues

- Depression

- Muscle weakness

- Joint pain

- Migraine

- Headaches

- Lethargy

- Inability to concentrate

- Cloudy thinking

- Cravings for food you are allergic to

The symptoms above may seem minor, but they are all reactions to food allergy.

Is There a Way to Test for Food Sensitivity?

You can ask your doctor to order a blood test to help identify your sensitivity level to most common culprits. However, there are some who claim that the results of the test is not reliable, particularly the low to moderate scores. Regardless, it's a good starting point. You will have a list of specific foods that you can monitor for any reactions or try eliminating from your diet. If you have multiple food allergies, which is quite likely, a blood test is an easiest and fastest way to determine which foods they are.

If you do not have a doctor, you can order a lab test for food sensitivity directly from certain laboratories. This test will not be cheap, but you will able to get the results after 7 days after the lab receives your sample. You can also order a one-on-one phone consultation with a medical doctor to go over your results.

If you decide to self-diagnose, you can follow an elimination diet designed to identify many of the most common food sensitives quickly while maintaining a positive focus on building up the food list that you are not reactive to help treat and recover from adrenal fatigue. The book "The Plan" by LynGenet Recitas is also a very helpful reading.

Is There a Cure for Food Allergies?

Fortunately, it is possible to reverse some of the IgG delayed food allergies. The vital step when you have allergies to multiple foods is to begin eliminating the ones on your sensitivity list for about 2-3 months – it can take that long to clear all the allergens in your system. During this period, you should take a good probiotic to help repopulate your intestinal tract with beneficial bacteria to aid digestion. You can also drink Aloe Vera juice, which is known to have useful healing properties for the intestinal tract. If your food allergies have caused overgrowth of Candida yeast in your gut, then this is also the time to cure them as well.

After the cleansing and healing time, you can begin reintroducing the foods you have eliminated one at a time, starting with offenders with the lowest score indicated in your test result.

After the resting period, it will be obvious which foods cause a particular reaction. It is possible that many of the foods that you are sensitive to can be tolerated in infrequent or small amounts.

Start a journal noting each food you try to reintroduce in your diet. If you experience no reaction during the first day, try that food for the next day. If you have no reaction, then have more on the third day. After that, wait for four days before trying the next lowest score on your sensitivity list, following the same method. Keep in mind that if you have a reaction, you should stop trying that food.

Now that you have a complete idea on how to start your adrenal fatigue treatment and recovery, make the lifestyle changes that will suit your needs. The first step for a healthier you is to take charge of your health.

Final Words

Thank you again for purchasing this book! I really hope this book is able to help you.

The next step is for you to **join our email newsletter** to receive updates on any upcoming new book releases or promotions. You can sign-up for free and as a bonus, you will also receive our "*7 Fitness Mistakes You Don't Know You're Making*" book! This bonus book breaks down many of the most common fitness mistakes and will demystify many of the complexities and science of getting into shape. Having all this fitness knowledge and science organized into an actionable step-by-step book will help you get started in the right direction in your fitness journey! To join our free email newsletter and grab your free book, please visit the link and signup: **www.hmwpublishing.com/gift**

Finally, if you enjoyed this book, then I would like to ask you for a favor, would you be kind enough to leave a review for this book? It would be greatly appreciated!

Thank you and good luck in your journey!

About the Co-Author

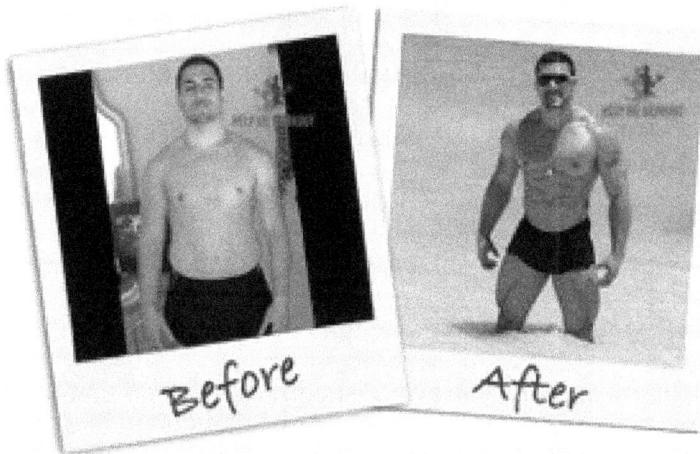

Before   After

My name is George Kaplo; I'm a certified personal trainer from Montreal, Canada. I'll start off by saying I'm not the biggest guy you will ever meet and this has never really been my goal. In fact, I started working out to overcome my biggest insecurity when I was younger, which was my self-confidence. This was due to my height measuring only 5 foot 5 inches (168cm), it pushed me down to attempt anything I ever wanted to achieve in life. You may be going through some challenges right now, or you may simply want to get fit, and I can certainly relate.

For me personally, I was always kind of interested in the

health & fitness world and wanted to gain some muscle due to the numerous bullying in my teenage years about my height and my overweight body. I figured I couldn't do anything about my height, but I sure can do something about how my body looked like. This was the beginning of my transformation journey. I had no idea where to start, but I just got started. I felt worried and afraid at times that other people would make fun of me for doing the exercises the wrong way. I always wished I had a friend that was next to me who was knowledgeable enough to help me get started and "show me the ropes."

After a lot of work, studying and countless trial and errors. Some people began to notice how I was getting more fit and how I was starting to form a keen interest in the topic. This led many friends and new faces to come to me and ask me for fitness advice. At first, it seemed odd when people asked me to help them get in shape. But what kept me going is when they started to see changes in their own body and told me it's the first time that they saw real results! From there, more people kept coming to me, and it made me realize after so much reading and studying in this field that it did help me but it also allowed me to help others. I'm now a fully certified personal trainer and have trained numerous clients to date who have achieved amazing results.

Today, my brother Alex Kaplo (also a Certified Personal Trainer) and I own & operate this publishing venture, where we bring passionate and expert authors to write about health and fitness topics. We also run an online fitness website "HelpMeWorkout.com" and I would love to connect with by inviting you to visit the website on the following page and signing up to our e-mail newsletter (you will even get a free book).

Last but not least, if you are in the position I was once in and you want some guidance, don't hesitate and ask... I'll be there to help you out!

Your friend and coach,

George Kaplo
Certified Personal Trainer

Download another book for Free

I want to thank you for purchasing this book and offer you another book (just as long and valuable as this book), "Health & Fitness Mistakes You Don't Know You're Making", completely free.

Visit the link below to signup and receive it:

www.hmwpublishing.com/gift

In this book, I will break down the most common health & fitness mistakes, you are probably committing right now, and I will reveal how you can easily get in the best shape of your life!

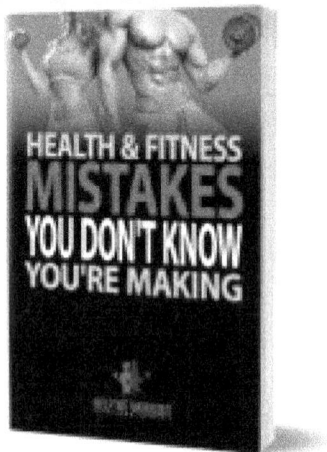

In addition to this valuable gift, you will also have an opportunity to get our new books for free, enter giveaways, and receive other valuable emails from me. Again, visit the link to sign up:

www.hmwpublishing.com/gift

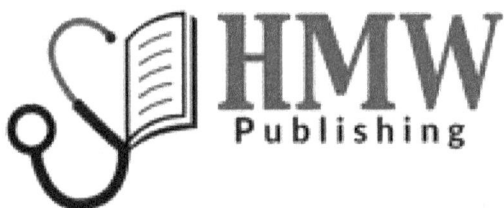

For more great books visit:

HMWPublishing.com